An Easy Way To Understand Heart Disease High Blood Pressure Stroke

Also By Brian B Jacques

His very popular Series of Mini-Health Books includes:

- An Easy Way To Understand Eczema and Psoriasis
- An Easy Way To Understand Stress and Depression
- An Easy Way To Understand Vitamins and Minerals
- An Easy Way To Understand Parasites, Worms, Candida, Constipation & Detoxing
- An Easy Way To Understand Crohn's Disease and IBD
- An Easy Way To Understand Body Building For Men And Women
- An Easy Way To Understand Alzheimer's Disease
- An Easy Way To Understand Herpes
- An Easy Way To Understand Parkinson's Disease
- An Easy Way To Understand Autism
- An Easy Way To Understand Fibromyalgia
- An Easy Way To Understand Your Body Systems
- An Easy Way To Understand Erectile Dysfunction
- An Easy Way To Understand Heart Disease, High Blood Pressure & Stroke
- An Easy Way To Understand Detoxing For Men & Women
- An Easy Way To Understand Diabetic Neuropathy
- An Easy Way To Understand Aromatherapy & Essential Oils
- Herbs For Healing
- How To Lose Weight After 40
- How To Lose Weight And Maintain Your Ideal Weight Permanently
- Amino Acids & Enzymes—What Are They & Why Do You Need Them
- The Little A–Z Dictionary of Herbal Remedies
- The Magic Of Vitamins & Minerals
- Effective Methods To Stop Smoking
- Eat Wholefoods And Take Supplements—The Ultimate Lifestyle Guide
- Stress Busters Adult Coloring Book
- An Easy Way To Understand ADHD For Children And Adults

An Easy Way To Understand Heart Disease High Blood Pressure Stroke

Brian B Jacques

Wisdom For Life Media

Publisher: Wisdom For Life Media.

While they have made every effort to verify the information provided in this publication, neither the author nor the publisher assumes any responsibility for errors in, omissions from, or different interpretation of the subject matter.

The information herein may be subject to varying laws, regulations, and practices in different areas, states and countries. The purchaser or reader assumes all responsibility for use of the information.

All information included within this book is for educational purposes only. The author and publishers do not attempt to diagnose or treat any medical conditions, be it to do with health, diet or exercise.

If you consider that you have any kind of medical condition, then, you should consult a qualified medical practitioner or doctor or qualified naturopathic doctor before starting any herbal, vitamin and/or mineral program or supplement regime, exercise or health training program or diet suggested in this book.

This book is not intended for anyone under the age of 18 years, nor is it intended for breast feeding or pregnant women, underweight people or anyone with eating disorders or a health condition that requires special diets or medical treatment.

The author and publishers disclaim any liability for any loss however caused by anyone using the information contained in this book.

ISBN - 9798492849535

Published in The United States of America.

*"Education is the kindling of a flame,
not the filling of a vessel."—Socrates*

Contents

Acknowledgment

To the many people I have come into contact with throughout my life, whose belief in me has made everything possible and worthwhile.

Introduction

The Biggest Mass Killer In The US

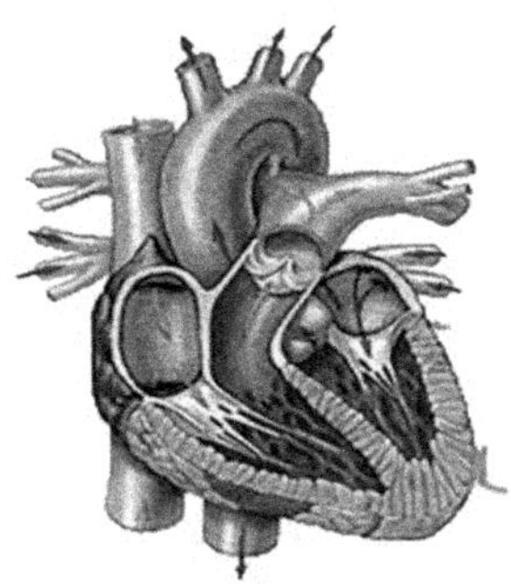

Coronary Heart Disease—or CHD for short—kills more people in the United States than any other disease. The second biggest killer is cancer (of all forms). Coronary Heart Disease claims the life of someone every 34 seconds.

I have included reference tables at the back of this book which show mortality statistics for the top ten causes of death in the four main countries whose citizens purchase my health books. These are: the US, Canada, part of the UK (England and Wales) and Australia.

These statistics always lag a few years behind for some reason, but they give a good insight into a nation's health, and what diseases are the main causes of death in each country. If you wish to obtain further information, then all the statistics you require are available for free download from each country's statistics organization's website.

Interestingly, the US still shows the highest death rates for heart disease. However, Canada, Australia and England and Wales now show cancer (of all forms) as being the main cause of death.

In some ways this is hardly surprising as the amount of publicity (and money) devoted to reducing heart disease in Canada, Australia and England and Wales has certainly been successful, but, the rates of cancer deaths still give cause for concern.

And when you consider the amount of money that goes into cancer research, you would think that more progress would have been made to reduce the death rate of this devastating disease. Still, there are over 200 types of cancer so it is a huge issue.

So, back to this book and heart disease.

Obviously the risk of a heart attack increases as you get older, but you can still help prevent one.

CHD happens when your blood supply gets blocked by an accumulation of fatty plaques called atheroma in your coronary arteries. What happens is that over time these fatty substances build up in a process known as atherosclerosis. When these arteries get clogged up the blood can't get through to your heart. The result is chest pains—or angina. There are around 10 million people with this condition in the US.

When the vessels become completely blocked that's when you have a heart attack or to give it its technical name myocardial infarction.

There's another associated problem. Narrowing of arteries in the neck can cause loss of blood supply to the brain and this leads to a stroke, which can be catastrophic affecting both your physical and mental capacities. We'll look at this in much more detail later.

A stroke, heart attack, angina and circulatory disease are all known as cardiovascular diseases or CVD.

Yet there are plenty of ways you can change your lifestyle to reduce the likelihood of a heart attack. If you already suffer from heart problems, there's still a lot you can do to reduce the risk of it getting any worse.

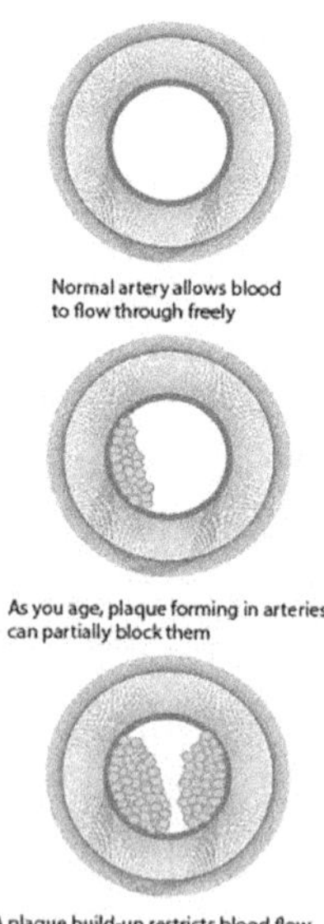

Chapter 1

Types of Heart Disease

Cardiomyopathy

This term means heart muscle disease and it's what happens when the main heart muscle deteriorates and there can be a number of reasons for this. It can be linked to alcohol, congenital heart disease and a wide variety of other conditions. People with this type of CHD risk sudden cardiac death.

Ischemic heart disease

Ischemic heart disease is a disease characterized by reduced blood supply to the heart. It is the most common cause of death in most western countries.

Ischemia means a "reduced blood supply".

The coronary arteries purpose is to supply blood to the heart muscle and where no alternative blood supply exists, a blockage in the coronary arteries occurs which reduces the supply of blood to the heart muscle. Most cases of ischemic heart disease are caused by atherosclerosis, usually present even when the artery lumens appear normal by angiography.

In the Initial stages there is a sudden severe narrowing or closure of either the large coronary arteries and/or of coronary artery end branches by debris showering downstream in the flowing blood. It is usually felt as angina, especially if a large area is affected.

The narrowing or closure is mainly caused by the covering of atheromatous plaques within the wall of the artery rupturing, in turn leading to a heart attack. A heart attack causes damage to the heart muscle by cutting off its blood supply.

Heart failure

Sometimes called congestive heart or cardiac failure, this is a condition resulting from any disorder which stops the heart from filling with or pumping enough blood through the body.

Hypertensive heart disease

This is a disease which is caused by high blood pressure especially when you find it in localized areas.

Inflammatory heart disease

This is what happens when the muscle in the heart or the tissues surrounding it become inflamed. Inflammation of the heart muscle itself is known as myocarditis. Endocarditis is an inflammation of the inner layer of the heart, most commonly the heart valves.

Valvular heart disease

This is when one or more of the valves in the heart become diseased. The technical terms for the right-sided valves are the tricuspid and pulmonic valves. On the left they're known as the mitral and aortic valves.

Symptoms of Angina

The main symptoms of angina are a pain or tightness in the middle of your chest or heaviness. But you might also find it in your arms (particularly your left) as well as your face, jaw, abdomen or back. It normally happens after sudden exertion like climbing stairs or rushing to catch a plane. But it's also brought on by cold weather, when you've eaten a big meal or when you're feeling stressed.

There are other symptoms, too, but the problem we face is that these could be linked to other medical conditions:

- Sudden breathlessness even when you're not exerting yourself.
- Rapid palpitations of the heart sometimes lasting several hours or days. It may be accompanied by chest pains, dizziness or breathlessness.
- Fainting.
- Retaining fluid or puffiness in the tissues of your legs, lungs, ankles or abdomen. This is known as edema.
- When your fingernails or lips have a bluish tinge because of too little oxygen in the blood. This is called cyanosis.
- Fatigue. But here we have to be careful because it can also signal all sorts of other conditions such as depression.

Chapter 2

So Who Is At Risk?

Despite decades of research there is still no definitive answer as to what actually causes CHD. What is known is that there are key risk factors which can significantly increase your chances of developing heart disease. Unfortunately there is nothing you can do about some of them, such as: age, ethnic background or gender.

But with others such as smoking, diet and exercise you certainly can. Keeping down your blood pressure and cholesterol intake, stopping smoking, reducing alcohol intake, getting more exercise and reducing your weight can all help.

Age

It is well proven that your chances of developing CHD increase as you get older. Atherosclerosis (the build-up of fatty plaque in your arteries) takes a long time to develop. Arteries naturally become a lot less flexible the older you get and this leads to a greater risk of hypertension (high blood pressure.)

Gender

Traditionally we've looked on CHD as very much a men's problem but it also kills more women than any other disease. During a woman's reproductive years her sex hormone estrogen protects against CHD because it not only balances the amount of fats in the blood but it also helps keep the heart arteries elastic. But after the menopause or when women have had a hysterectomy, this natural form of protection can vanish.

Women who use oral contraceptives run a bigger risk of blood clotting problems which can lead to thrombosis or a heart attack. It's only a small risk but it increases if you smoke.

Genes

Your genetic make-up may make you more prone to heart problems. If you've got a family history where members have had high cholesterol or blood pressure, you may run a greater risk.

Ethnic background

African Americans or Asian people run a greater risk of heart attacks but there are different risk factors affecting these groups of people. Asian people have a bigger chance of developing diabetes which is a key factor. African Americans, on the other hand, are more likely to suffer from high blood pressure.

Diabetes

People suffering from diabetes are three times more likely to develop CHD than those who don't. And there is another complication here. Since diabetes can affect the nerves which send out pain, you may have a painless angina or a heart attack. This is especially dangerous because people receive no warning that there are problems going on in their hearts and don't seek any help.

Chapter 3

Why Prevention is Better Than Cure

Few people can be unaware that making a major effort to tame America's biggest killer has become one of the government's main priorities over the past few years. And the figures show that the battle is being won—slowly. There's been lots of publicity about all the things you can and should do to cut down on the risks.

It's a bit of a cliché that prevention is better than cure. Yet some people fail to do anything at all until a crisis develops. Sometimes it takes a heart attack for people to change their lifestyle and habits.

So what are the key weapons you've got to keep heart disease at bay?

Some Good Reasons Why You Should Stop Smoking

If you don't smoke, then you can skip this section. On the other hand, if you do smoke, then this section may give you a good reason to quit. We all know that smoking is an addiction. And once you start, it is difficult to stop. The body does crave nicotine, but interestingly, it leaves the bloodstream 48 hours after smoking your final cigarette. But what about the addiction? It can be termed as physical and psychological in that it can be seen as helping with weight loss, to reduce stress and / or nervous habits as well as being a social habit.

So why should you stop smoking? To start with there are very good health reasons to stop. Smoking has been linked to an increased incidence of lung cancer as well as an increased risk of heart disease, stroke and hypertension (high blood pressure).

Therefore this is perhaps the single most important thing you can do to reduce the risk of suffering from these serious health issues. Reducing this risk has been one of the government's key measures to improve the nation's health. It's now banned nearly everywhere. You can't switch on the TV without adverts urging you to stop and offering ways to help. There's a lot of other advice available, too.

So why is smoking so dangerous? For a start the chemicals in tobacco smoke make the heart work a lot faster. Apart from the smoke containing various poisons it also affects the blood flow and damages the lining of arteries so that fatty substances build up and further slow-down blood-flow.

There is also the social aspect as well. Many people these days do not particularly like to be associated with someone who smokes. Then there is the secondary smoke aspect as well. If you do not smoke, but live or associate with someone who does, then it is as if you are smoking yourself as well by the very fact that you are inhaling the smoke from the other person. If your partner smokes in the house or car, then the effects of the smoke will get into the clothes you are wearing, carpets, window drapes, upholstery and any other type of fabric. This is called third hand smoking. Both the second and third hand types of smoking are as deadly as the first type.

So let us list some of the health reasons why you should stop smoking. You can probably think of several other reasons not listed here which are applicable to your situation.

As mentioned above, your health is certainly adversely affected by the fact that you smoke. Your lungs can be severely damaged. The bronchioles and bronchiole tree can become inflamed and swollen which impacts your ability to breathe in adequate amounts of oxygen. Additionally, if you smoke for any length of time, then your lungs with become coated with a tar-like substance which can have an even more damaging effect on your lungs ability to perform adequately.

When the lungs cells become swollen, they secrete a liquid which is associated with wheezing when you breathe, as well as being associated with "smokers cough".

Did you realize that each cigarette you smoke contains over 100 carcinogenic chemicals and toxic substances that have the effect of changing the chemical make-up of your body?

Breathing in cigarette smoke also means that you are breathing in carbon monoxide. This affects your hemoglobin as carbon monoxide takes up the space normally taken by oxygen. Therefore as a result, you don't have enough oxygen which means you will experience fatigue.

I mentioned lung cancer previously; smoking makes you more at risk for this deadly disease by decreasing your ability to breathe properly which is caused by the constant inflammation of the lungs cells.

You are also at greater risk of increased hypertension (blood pressure). This puts you at a greater risk of having a heart attack or stroke. Statistics show that you are more susceptible to these conditions than a non-smoker no matter what your age, sex or racial origins.

Emphysema is another serious condition associated with smoking.

There are also social issues as well which a smoker should consider; possibly the most important is that your loved one is in all probability concerned that you will damage your health and die of a smoking related disease before your time.

Smoking is a dirty habit which makes your clothes smell as well as your hair and breath. Not forgetting all the ash and cigarette ends that are left behind.

Imagine someone wanting to kiss you. It must be like kissing a smelly ashtray.

Think of your home. Smoking changes the color of the paint, especially on the ceiling which often becomes a yellow color. The paint on the walls suffers too as well as making the material on the window drapes, sofa and chairs smell as well.

Have you noticed that smoking is now not allowed in many public places and that some cities and states are considering banning smoking in the street as well?

Many employers and insurance companies take a dim view of anyone who smokes. It is a known fact that smokers have a higher risk of developing a serious illness than non-smokers. Insurance companies charge a higher insurance rate for anyone who smokes. Additionally employers who have a lower number of employees who smoke pay a lower insurance rate.

Cigarette smoking is not a cheap habit anymore. And while what you spend each week may seem insignificant, over a full year it really adds up. If you quit, then the money you save could probably pay for a great vacation somewhere, or you might like to treat your partner to a new wardrobe of clothes, or do something special for yourself.

Moving on to the psychological aspects: smoking cigarettes does not reduce your stress levels. In fact nicotine makes your body work harder instead.

In fact if you use cigarettes for stress reduction, you will find that it does not work in all situations which could leave you vulnerable and possibly unable to cope.

It is strange how you become reliant on a product that in all probability will ultimately kill you, all in the name of appearing "cool" and kidding yourself that it helps reduce your stress levels.

In the above I have given you a few reasons why it is a good idea to quit smoking. I am sure that if you think about it you will come up with many more reasons to quit that will fit your particular circumstances. The day you stop smoking is the day that your body will start to make a recovery from all the damage that you have inflicted upon it. So why not make today the day you decide to make a fundamental change for the better.

Exercise

Seven out of ten people in the United States don't get enough exercise. You don't have to climb a mountain or run a marathon. You don't even have to join a gym. Just 30 minutes exercise a day can make big improvements to your health. And it doesn't have to be a chore. It can actually be fun.

Therefore for exercise "regular" is what reaps the results. Research repeatedly shows that people who participate in regular physical activity are far healthier compared to those, who do not. They are even more likely to maintain a healthy weight.

Both men and women lose about a third of a pound of muscle mass each year after 40 years of age. Muscle is what burns the calories we eat, so less muscle mass means that fewer calories will be burned and more will be stored, that leads to greater susceptibility towards overweight, obesity, heart disease, diabetes and hypertension (high blood pressure).

Almost 79 million Americans are classed as being obese, which computes into an annual cost of $147 billion in healthcare and associated costs. Being obese will put an extra strain on your heart, therefore, starting a mild exercise program and building this up into a more substantial exercise regime can be very beneficial to your overall health.

Part of the secret to keeping weight in check is to keep as much muscle as you possibly can, and exercise is definitely the answer to this. There is no hard and fast rule to what exercise should be adopted. Any exercise, any fitness regime is good as long as you enjoy doing it, and can carry it on for a lifetime.

Remember it is important to burn more calories than you eat. While writing this, I researched a lot of different exercise programs. There was only one answer – whatever the exercise, it is important to just "do it"!

Strength and endurance exercises are considered cornerstones of a healthy body. Strength exercises means working the muscles with weights. This keeps muscles intact and reduces the muscle loss due to aging. For best results to maintain muscle mass, work weights with the large muscle groups such as those in the back, abdomen and thighs. These exercises also keep calcium in the bones which helps keep them strong.

On the other hand endurance exercises strengthen the heart and other muscles in the body. This group of exercises includes swimming, walking and dancing. It helps with efficient flow of blood and oxygen to the cells. These exercises help to burn the fat reserves. So a combination of both exercises can be beneficial.

Experts recommend that strength training exercises should be done at least twice a week for 15 minutes or more. Building muscles can be done either by using large machines or inexpensive hand and leg weights, by calisthenics or even lifting food cans!

For the endurance exercise group you should burn 300 calories every day. At this level you can lose weight and get rid of fat easily. This can be achieved by doing 30 minutes of cross country skiing or aerobics or 45 minutes of bike riding, swimming or walking.

Walking doesn't require any special fitness equipment, but it uses all the major muscle groups in the lower back, buttocks and legs. Because walking involves large muscles, elevation of the heart rate into a cardiovascular training zone is easy; hence a person then burns more calories. All that is needed is to put on a pair of shoes and go. It is not necessary to walk miles; even short walks count, as long as you do enough of them throughout the day.

According to the *American College of Sports Medicine*, effective health gains come from moderate-intensity physical activity accumulated throughout the day in 10-minute bouts. Health gains can include lower blood pressure, weight loss and overall improved disease management.

In studies exploring long-term weight loss (five years or longer), a common element of success was accumulating 200 or more minutes of moderate intensity exercise per week. Even 10 minute bouts of walking will count towards the total.

How much exercise does it take to reach 200 minutes per week? Only about 30 minutes each day. An easy way to start a walking program is to use a pedometer and take the 10,000 step challenge. A pedometer is a device about the size of a pager that typically attaches to a belt or waistband. It is designed primarily to count steps. Pedometers are capable of recording any weight-bearing activity you do such as walking, jogging or running.

According to Australian research if you walk less than 5,000 steps a day, you're sedentary. If you walk between 5,000 and 10,000 steps, you're somewhat active and if you walk more than 10,000 steps, you're active. This isn't to diminish your activity rating if you're cycling, rowing or swimming (which pedometers can't account for), but if you're not, then this rating could apply to you.

Walking is both physically and psychologically rewarding. Instead of sitting on a couch thinking over issues, it is always better to go out in a park and think while walking. This way you won't only burn calories; you will feel better as well.

Walking needs no aim! You can go out walking on your own, with a family member or even with the dog. Walk, walk and walk if it is weight you want to lose.

So in short, for a perfect walk routine, keep the following points in mind:

- 30-60 minutes at 50-70% of your maximum heart rate are recommended.
- Start with walking at an easy pace for 5-10 minutes.
- Stop and do some stretches and flexibility exercises.

- Walk at your target heart rate for 30-60 minutes.
- Cool down at a slower pace for 5 minutes.
- Finish with some gentle stretches.
- For longer walks, walk 30-60 minutes at your target heart rate and slow a bit to complete 90 or 120 minutes at a comfortable pace.

No matter what exercise you opt to do there are certain common guidelines for each of them. Never exert yourself. Exertion won't do you any good it will only harm your body and will lower your tolerance. Try starting a gradual pattern for your exercise regime.

Start in a minimal and effortless way, and when your body gets used to this, move to the next level. Similarly, at every session do not abruptly stop the exercise, this may cause harm to your heart and circulatory system. It is always best to taper the session. Starting with a warm up session is important, ending gradually is also very important too. Bring your heartbeat almost back to normal and then stop.

Exercising depends on many factors including age, weight and gender. Some exercises are not meant for certain age groups due to physical limitations. Similarly, women also have a few restrictions due to their body type and are unable to do extremely tough exercises that men can do.

Try doing any exercise, but do not exert yourself and if your body responds well to it then you can carry on with the same exercise; otherwise you should try something else.

There are several options in both strength training and endurance exercises, so you can choose any other from the same group. For example walking and jogging are both in the same strength training group. Walking is good for everyone, at any age, whatever weight you currently are. But jogging is not good for people over 35 years of age who have increased body weight, as it will put extra strain on the heart.

Regular exercise also has another benefit for your heart. It helps to control your weight which is another crucial factor in helping prevent CHD. On top of that you'll feel and probably look a lot better.

Eating and drinking

Another cliché is, "You are what you eat." And it's absolutely true. Many people have absolutely awful diets and that's why those who eat deep fried foods tend not to reach old age. Fresh food is always better than processed because for a start it has a lot less salt, which is one substance to avoid if you want to keep a healthy heart.

Alongside salt, fatty foods are also a killer. There's a huge stack of evidence to show that eating a low fat diet cuts the amount of cholesterol in your system which reduces the risks for CHD. In particular, many doctors advise reducing those saturated fats you get in burgers, meat, dairy products, cakes and cookies.

Chapter 4

Extra Fats: How It Impacts On the Whole Body And Your Health

More Than Meets the Eye

Almost all of us give ourselves a little extra time in front of the mirror every morning, either praising our good body shape or loathing the hideous bulging fat. No one ever desires to be overweight or obese. Gaining a few pounds for extra curves is one thing, but having excess fat cells is something else.

Fat cells or adipocytes are specialized cells that are capable of storing fats within themselves, which can be used as the energy source. Adipocytes are usually placed in bunches making up the tissue; the adipose tissue. Adipose tissue can be divided into two types: white adipose tissue (WAT) and brown adipose tissue (BAT), which are also known as white fat and brown fat, respectively. White fat is basically responsible for weight gain and obesity.

An average adult has 30 billion fat cells with a weight of 30 pounds or 13.5 kilograms. And the surprising part is when a person is putting on weight, these cells increase in size by up to four times their original size and weight, and then they divide! That means up to 120 pounds, approximately 54 kilograms of total fat can be stored in the original number of cells. The unfortunate thing for those watching their weight is that these cells are capable of growing back in size with excess fat, the moment you stop taking care of your diet.

The surprising fact is that 68% of the population is unaware of the side effects of overweight or obesity. For them it is only a matter of appearance. But in actual fact this is a condition where "beauty lies in the eyes of the beholder". It is also not an effective excuse for being fat.

Overweight and obesity are health conditions in their own right. But the story doesn't end here. Both these conditions affect multiple organs, and unfortunately these organs have to pay the price. Let's have a look at some vital organs and the effects excess body weight has on them.

Our circulatory system basically comprises the heart and vascular bundles (including arteries, veins and capillaries). When there is excess fat, cholesterol levels increase, resulting in the deposition of cholesterol in the lumens of arteries, veins and capillaries. The deposition of cholesterol provides resistance in the pumping of blood, which slows down the circulation along with pressure on the heart to pump more vigorously. According to a study each extra one pound, approximately 500 grams of fat requires an estimated 200 miles of new capillary networks to do the basic job.

The blocked capillaries may also cause eyesight damage by the bursting of tiny capillaries, causing damage to sensitive nerve tissue, which may even lead to blindness.

Being overweight or obese increases the prevalence of most cardiovascular risk factors. The disturbed circulatory system will not only affect the heart and blood vessels but it also affects other organs indirectly through hypertension (high blood pressure). It results not only in an increase in heart rate and blood volume, but also in an increased systolic and diastolic blood pressure. This can cause severe damage to the heart along with stroke, bursting blood vessels, dizziness, headache, fatigue, and insomnia.

Obesity increases the risk for the development of type II Diabetes. Unfortunately, medications used for hyperglycemia and hypertension, including sulphonylureas, insulin and beta-blockers, are themselves associated with weight gain. Hence, it becomes like a never ending vicious circle.

Renal functions are also impaired by the effects of excess weight on the kidneys. People with known renal disease have marked high risks for progressive renal function loss due to overweight. Moreover poor circulation may also affect renal functions that can lead to renal failure. The mechanism responsible for the renal damage caused by obesity has not been established but there is evidence suggesting that this might be related to both hormonal changes as well as low-grade inflammation.

Being overweight or obese can lead to a fatty Liver. Nonalcoholic fatty liver disease (NAFLD) refers to a wide spectrum of liver diseases ranging from the most common, fatty liver (accumulation of fat in the liver, also known as steatosis), to cirrhosis (irreversible, advanced scarring of the liver as a result of chronic inflammation of the liver).

All of the stages of nonalcoholic fatty liver disease are now believed to be due to insulin resistance, a condition closely associated with overweight and obesity. In fact, the BMI (Body Mass Index — measures how healthy your weight is based on how tall you are) correlates with the degree of liver damage, that is, the greater the BMI the greater the liver damage. You can find excellent BMI tables on the Internet to work out your own BMI.

Increased weight will also affect the gallbladder. There are increased chances of blocked bile ducts, which may not only impair fat digestion but can also form gall stones, which are extremely painful and agitating.

Being overweight not only affects vital organs it also has an impact on muscles and joints. There is a 40% increased risk for developing arthritis. Back pain, sprains and tiredness are usually associated issues with excess weight. Joints are also susceptible to inflammation, swelling, stiffness, pain, arthritis and joint degeneration. Similarly developing a hernia also has an increased prevalence in obese people.

Excess weight is also associated with hormone imbalances. Nearly 90% of obese women suffer from Polycystic Ovarian Syndrome (PCOS), a complex hormonal disorder that affects a woman's menstrual cycle, fertility and insulin production.

The estrogen hormone not only determines the fat deposition pattern in females but it may also increase the risk of high blood pressure, infertility and malignant growths. Growth hormone is also related to excess weight as it also affects metabolism. Researchers have found that growth hormone levels in obese people are lower than those in people of normal weight.

Obstructive sleep apnea (that is, interrupted breathing during sleeping) is more common in overweight people. Obesity is associated with a higher prevalence of asthma and severe bronchitis, as well as obesity hypoventilation syndrome and respiratory insufficiency.

According to *Centers for Disease Control and Prevention (CDC)* researchers, an estimated 300,000 American deaths a year are related to obesity. The risk of premature death rises with increasing weight. Even moderate weight gain (10 to 20 pounds for a person of average height) increases the risk of death, particularly among adults aged 30 to 64 years.

Apart from doing devastating physical damage, being overweight also affects the psychological health of the individual, which may also be linked to social and socio-economic issues.

Chapter 5

High Blood Pressure—The Silent Killer

What is normal blood pressure?

At some time most people have had their blood pressure checked when they have visited their doctor's office. Normal blood pressure is defined as two figures 120 over 80, or 120/80, or lower. This ideal blood pressure means that you have a lower risk of having heart disease or stroke.

Your blood pressure varies throughout the day and depends on whether you are anxious, stressed or have been exercising. So a one-off reading doesn't necessarily mean that you've got high blood pressure. So the best way is to take a number of readings at different times when you are relaxed. This could be over several weeks or even months. Also remember that you will get a different reading from the left arm and the right arm. So it is an idea to use the arm which consistently gives the highest reading.

High blood pressure—or hypertension—increases your chances of a heart attack or stroke. The higher your blood pressure the higher the risk.

Elevated blood pressure is more common in older people than it is in younger people.

How is it measured?

Blood pressure is measured in something called millimeters of mercury (mmHg) and two figures are assessed such as 140 over 90. The first number is the pressure in the arteries when the heart contracts called the systolic pressure. The second is the pressure when the heart rests between beats and is known as the diastolic pressure.

What Causes High Blood Pressure

Often there is no single cause in most people who develop high blood pressure. However your lifestyle can put you more at risk of developing it if you:

- Are overweight
- Do not get enough exercise
- Don't eat enough fruit and vegetables

- Eat too much food containing saturated fat
- Eat too much salt
- Consume too much alcohol

There are several factors that can increase your risk of developing high blood pressure, factors over which you have no control. Some of these are:

- Age—as you get older, the lifestyle you have led previously can catch up with you with the result that your blood pressure can increase.
- Ethnic groups—people from South Asia and the African Caribbean cultures are at greater risk of developing high blood pressure.
- Genetics—if you have a family history of high blood pressure then you have a higher than average risk of developing high blood pressure.
- If you have certain medical conditions or take certain medications, this can raise your blood pressure levels significantly.

So Have I Got High Blood Pressure?

If your blood pressure is 120 over 80 (120/80) then you have a normal blood pressure and your goal will be to keep it at this reading, or aim to get it lower.

If your blood pressure is between 120 over 80 and 140 over 90 (120/80 – 140/90) your reading is normal, but a bit on the high side. You should aim to reduce it by making healthy choices to your diet and lifestyle.

If your blood pressure is over 140 over 90 (140/90) and it stays at this level for a number of weeks, then, you may have high blood pressure (another name for this is hypertension). You will need to consult your doctor for blood pressure reducing medication and you will also need to assess you diet and lifestyle.

However, some people whose blood pressure is between 120 over 80 and 140 over 90 (120/80-140/90) need to work at getting it lower if they are at risk of developing CVD, are diabetes sufferers and those with kidney or liver damage.

Your goal should be to keep your blood pressure in the normal range by carefully assessing your diet and lifestyle. It often doesn't take much to make changes that will have a very beneficial effect on your blood pressure. Remember, if you blood pressure rises, then, it will put you at greater risk of developing serious health conditions such as heart disease and stroke.

Some people are given or buy blood pressure monitors so they can keep track of their levels at home. This is because going to clinics automatically makes some people nervous, which can make their blood pressure rise.

Should I Get My Blood Pressure Checked

Most of the time high blood pressure doesn't actually throw up any symptoms. You might be completely unaware that you've got a problem—until you get it checked out. That means everyone should have a check every three to five years. In older people, those with diabetes or those who've had a previously high reading, it should be every year.

Over time high blood pressure may lead to a heart attack, stroke or kidney damage. It may also damage your arteries and put extra strain on your heart. You may also suffer from increased headaches, feel drowsy and have redness in your face. As a general rule, the greater your blood pressure, the higher the health risk you run.

What Causes It

Several factors can cause your blood pressure to rise such as stress, hormonal issues or a narrowing of the arteries caused by a build-up of plaque which makes it more difficult for blood to flow through easily. See the diagram on the following page.

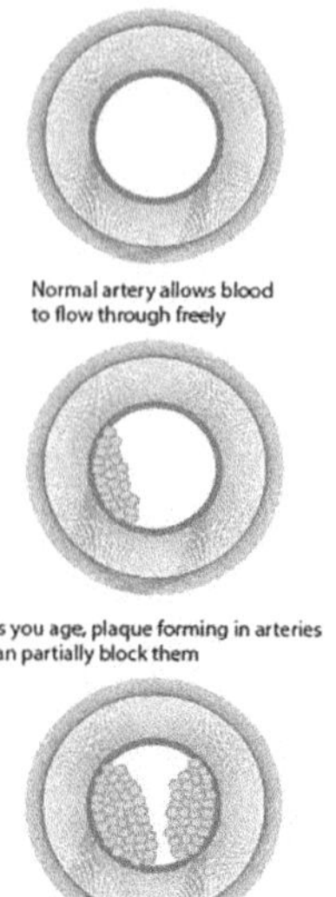

Normal artery allows blood to flow through freely

As you age, plaque forming in arteries can partially block them

A plaque build-up restricts blood flow which can lead to a heart attack or stroke

Who Is At Risk

High blood pressure is more common among certain groups of people:

- People with particular lifestyle factors who are overweight, eat a lot of food that is high in saturated fat, don't eat many fruits and vegetables, don't take much or any exercise, drink a lot of coffee or caffeine-rich drinks and who consume a lot of alcohol.
- Those with a family history of high blood pressure.
- Diabetes sufferers. Three out of ten people with Type 1 diabetes and more than half of people with Type 2 diabetes eventually develop high blood pressure.
- People of Afro-Caribbean or South Asian descent.
- People from the Indian sub-continent.
- People who work in a stressful environment

Chapter 6

How To Lower Your Blood Pressure

Remember, an unhealthy diet and lifestyle will raise your blood pressure over a period of time. The higher your blood pressure, the greater will be your risk of developing heart disease or having a stroke, as well as an increased risk of developing diabetes.

If doesn't always take a lot to bring your blood pressure down. You can start by looking at your diet and making more healthy choices, especially look at increasing your fiber intake.

Also assess how much exercise you do each day/week. Increasing your exercise levels will have a significant impact on lowering your blood pressure. It is always advisable to consult your doctor or health care provider before embarking on a diet program of any kind, or starting an exercise regime especially when you have not done hardly any exercise before.

Things to consider:

- Look at lowering your sodium (salt) intake. Excessive amounts of sodium will raise your blood pressure. There is "hidden sodium" in a lot of foods that you buy especially bread, breakfast cereals, and ready prepared meals. The picture on the box might look appetizing, but will it do your body any good? Finally, don't add sodium to food at the table. People who do this often do it out of habit rather than necessity. There is usually enough sodium in the food already without you adding more.
- Make sure you get your minimum of five servings of fruit and vegetables each day. You will get vitamins and minerals from fruit and vegetables as well as some fiber. But try not to overcook them, or you will destroy all the nutrients. Try to eat as much raw food as you can, to retain as much of the goodness as possible.
- Watch your weight. Being overweight puts extra strain on your heart and can lead to other health problems. Losing some weight will reduce your blood pressure. You can refer to two weight loss books I have published to the Kindle platform for some useful ideas. One way is to watch how many calories you consume each day, also switching to low fat and low calorie foods as well as **increasing** your exercise levels will all help.

- Watch your alcohol consumption. Drinking excess alcohol for long periods of time will increase your blood pressure.
- Get more exercise. Even a small amount of exercise done on a frequent basis will provide significant health benefits and will help to lower your blood pressure. If you can manage 30 minutes per day for five days each week that will provide even more benefits. Whatever exercise you do, start slowly and build up gradually. If you experience any discomfort, then discontinue immediately and seek medical advice. It is always best to discuss any exercise regime with your doctor before starting.

What Treatment Is Available

Sometimes doctors use a risk factor calculator to work out how likely high blood pressure is to cause problems. Things that will be taken into account include: age, sex, smoking, drinking, diet, weight, cholesterol level and the amount of exercise you take.

If you run the risk of developing CHD within the next ten years, then various preventive options will be discussed with you. These will include:

- Medication to lower your blood pressure if it's above 140/90.
- Medication to lower your cholesterol level. However, if you take a statin drug, then you will need to supplement with Co-Enzyme Q10 (CoQ10). CoQ10 is found in most cell of the body and is important for good heart health. Statins will destroy it.
- A daily dose of soluble aspirin (75mg) which cuts the risk of blood clots forming over the patches of atheroma (furred up arteries). The clots can cause a heart attack and/or a stroke.
- Changing your lifestyle by taking more exercise, stopping smoking, changing what you eat or losing weight. Losing weight can make an enormous difference. Your blood pressure can fall by 2.5/1.5 mmHg for every two pounds you lose. Previously inactive people who exercise five times a week can see systolic pressure fall by between 2 and 10. A healthier diet can reduce systolic pressure by up to 11.

Chapter 7

Stroke—What Is It

Basically a stroke is a "brain attack". It happens suddenly when the blood supply is cut off, stopping oxygen and vital nutrients. The effects are immediate. Brain cells can be damaged or destroyed. When they die this is known as a cerebral infarction.

Since the brain is our control box, body functions can be severely affected. For example, if the part of the brain which controls your limbs is affected, you won't be able to walk or use your arms.

But a stroke can also have a mental effect. It can affect the way you feel, think, communicate and learn.

Did you know?

- Approximately 795,000 Americans each year suffer a new or recurrent stroke. That means, on average, a stroke occurs every 40 seconds.
- Stroke kills more than 137,000 people each year. That's about 1 of every 18 deaths. It's the number four cause of death.
- On average, every 4 minutes someone dies of a stroke.
- About 40 percent of stroke deaths occur in males, and 60 percent in females.
- The 2006 stroke death rates per 100,000 of the population for specific groups were 41.7 for white males, 41.1 for white females, 67.7 for black males and 57.0 for black females.
- Americans will pay about $73.7 billion in 2010 for stroke-related medical costs and disability.

Types of Stroke

There are two types of stroke:

A blockage or ischemic stroke when a clot blocks an artery carrying blood to the brain. This could be caused by a cerebral thrombosis when a clot forms in the main artery to the brain. It could be a cerebral embolism caused by a clot, air bubble or fat globule formed somewhere else and carried to the brain. Or it could be a lacunar stroke when there's a blockage in the tiny blood vessels deep inside the brain.

A hemorrhagic stroke. This is when a blood vessel bursts causing bleeding into the brain. This could be caused by a blood vessel bursting within the brain (intracerebral hemorrhage). Or it could be when a blood vessel on the surface of the brain bleeds into the area between the brain and the skull (subarachnoid hemorrhage).

What Are The Symptoms

Strokes are sudden and often catastrophic. The symptoms include:

- Weakness, paralysis or numbness on one side of the body such as a drooping arm, a lowered eyelid or drooping mouth.
- Slurred speech or difficulty of understanding or finding words.
- Loss of sight or sudden blurred vision.
- Unsteadiness or confusion.
- A severe headache.

The FAST Test (Face, Arms, Speech, Time) may be used to determine whether someone has suffered a stroke or Transient Ischemic Attack (TIA), sometimes known as a mini-stroke. This happens when the blood supply to the brain is interrupted briefly.

- Facial weakness: Can the person smile? Has their mouth or an eye drooped?
- Arm weakness: Can the person raise both arms?
- Speech problems: Can the person speak clearly and understand what you say?
- Time to dial 9-1-1.

If the symptoms disappear after a few minutes or hours then it's probably a TIA rather than a stroke. The symptoms are very similar. But you should still treat it as a medical emergency because urgent assessment is needed. You need to see a doctor immediately or go to the ER at the hospital. A TIA can signal the possibility of a stroke in the future.

If when you are assessed the risk of a major stroke is high you should get an MRI brain scan within 24 hours. If the risk is low then this should take place within a week. If there is a possibility the blockage is caused by arteries at the front of the neck, then a scan of the carotid arteries will be performed. After all tests have been done, then it will be decided by your doctor whether surgery is needed.

Who Is Most At Risk

Strokes affect mainly older people but most of the risk factors are the same as for heart attacks.

If someone in your family has had a stroke, the risk of you having one is increased. That is because things like high blood pressure and cholesterol run in families.

Your ethnic background may also be a factor. People of Asian, African and Afro-Caribbean descent are at greater risk. Diabetes and high blood pressure tend to be higher among some ethnic groups.

The Effects

How you are affected depends entirely on which part of the brain has been damaged. Every stroke is different. For some people the effects are quite mild and last only a few minutes or hours. Other strokes may be much more serious and lead to permanent damage. Some brain cells are damaged and others are killed off. The damaged ones may recover as the swelling caused by the stroke subsides. It's possible that unaffected areas of the brain can take over those which have been damaged. It depends very much on the part of the brain affected, the seriousness of the attack and your health in general.

Most recovery takes place within a few months of having a stroke although in some cases it can take several years.

The right side of the brain controls the left side of the body and vice versa. So if the right side of your brain is damaged, it will affect the left side of your body. The left side of the brain controls things like speech, understanding, reading and writing. The right half is responsible for what are called perceptual skills such as making sense of what you see, hear and touch and also spatial skills like judging the speed, position, size and distance of objects.

Other Common Problems

In most people things improve as time goes on but in severe cases there's long-term disability. After a stroke you tend to get a number of lingering problems:

- Paralysis, weakness or clumsiness.
- Balance.
- Difficulty in swallowing. This affects around half of those who've suffered a stroke.

- Sleep and fatigue.
- Speech, language and writing. Difficulty in understanding what's been said is referred to as dysphasia.
- Eyesight.
- Bladder and bowel problems.
- Mood swings.
- Pain.
- Loss of sensation.

All in all then, each individual is definitely not powerless to dramatically reduce their risk of a heart attack, high blood pressure and stroke—even if it is in the genes. The situation is much better than it was even five years ago. Let's hope the next five years see similar improvements and more people living longer.

Chapter 8

Eat A Healthy Diet

- At least five and ideally seven to nine portions a day of fruit and vegetables.
- Most meals should be starch-based with cereals, whole-wheat bread, potatoes, rice and pasta plus fruit and vegetables.
- Reduce fatty foods such as fatty meats, cheeses, full-cream milk and butter. Go for low fat, mono or poly-unsaturated spreads.
- Processed foods and ready meals are often high in salt, sugar and saturated fat, in addition to transfats which are a big no no.
- Eat two or three portions of fish a week, one of which should be an oily fish such as mackerel, herring, kippers, pilchards, salmon or fresh tuna (not tinned).
- Choose lean meats or poultry such as chicken.
- Use vegetable oils such as sunflower, rapeseed or olive oil for frying.
- Go easy on the sodium (salt.)
- Healthy eating can lower cholesterol and reduce weight. A diet with plenty of vitamins, minerals, nutrients and fiber can help stave off other diseases.
- These days the quantities of salt and fats are shown on most food product labeling so it's easy to check what you are eating. In addition the government has introduced an "eat five a day" promotion. This information is also often included on food labels.

The USDA has produced a successor to the Food Guide Pyramid called "*Choose My Plate*" to help with your dietary requirements. This encourages you to choose a variety of foods from the main food groups which are:

- Fruits and vegetables
- Bread, cereals, pasta and potatoes
- Meat, fish and different types of protein (animal and vegetable derived)
- Dairy products such as milk, cheese and yoghurt
- Fats and oils (use these sparingly)

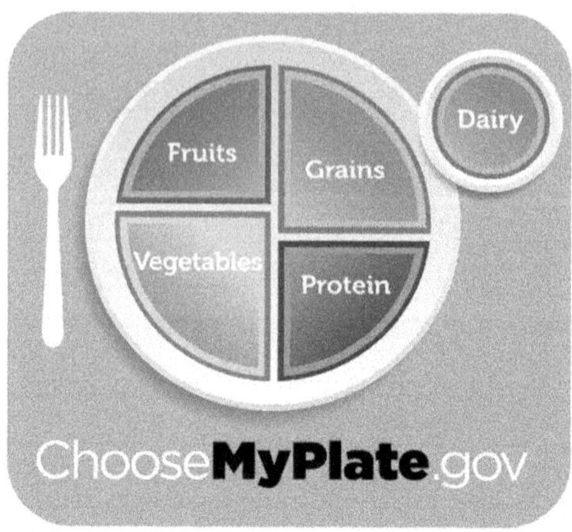

Copyright USDA Center for Nutrition Policy and Promotion.
www.choosemyplate.gov

Let us not forget fiber! Fiber plays an important role in reducing cholesterol and high blood pressure as well as helping to protect your heart and in stroke prevention. Foods high in fiber help to control blood fat levels. Sadly, the Western diet is often lacking in fiber and the consequences of this are seen in the statistics of a high rate of death from heart disease and stroke.

Good sources of fiber are: wholegrain cereals, whole wheat bread, whole wheat pasta, porridge oats, brown rice and couscous; as well as beans and lentils.

In my two books on vitamins and minerals which are available on the Amazon platform, I explained what these important nutrients do and the various functions they perform in the human body. Also, I explained how many of these are destroyed in food processing, food preparation, during storage and cooking.

Reducing the amount of alcohol you drink can also play an important part. Referring to the *Dietary Guidelines for Americans,* moderate alcohol consumption is defined as having up to 1 drink per day for women and up to 2 drinks per day for men. This definition is referring to the amount consumed on any single day and is not intended as an average over several days. The Dietary Guidelines also say that it is not recommended that anyone begin drinking or drink more frequently on the basis of potential health benefits because moderate alcohol intake is also associated with an increased risk of breast cancer, violence, drowning, and injuries from falls and motor vehicle accidents.

Watch your weight

Since World War II the US has tended to become a nation of overweight people and as evidence, there is now an alarming level of obesity especially among children who live on pizzas and convenience food. The more weight you are carrying around, the greater strain it puts on your heart. It also increases your chances of getting diabetes, which has a detrimental effect on your heart.

A lot of people want to lose weight but find it very difficult to do so. The temptations of chocolate, fast foods and other things which make you put on weight are all around us. But it's not rocket science.

But you should also reduce the amount you eat. It depends to a large extent on what you do. Someone with a physically demanding job normally needs to eat more than a secretary. After all, you really don't need 5,000 calories a day if you're sitting in an office. Men generally need more food than women. It's difficult to generalize because it does depend on your age, height, occupation and other factors, but the recommended minimum calorie intake is 1200 for women and 1800 for men.

The US weight loss industry is worth hundreds of millions of dollars a year. TV programs and magazines are crammed with advice (much of it plain nonsense) about how to lose weight. And there are hundreds of different and often trendy dieting methods from Atkins to eating nothing but fruit. As a health researcher, I sometimes feel rather skeptical about many of the claims of losing 40 pounds in five weeks. And you have to ask yourself if the claims made for many of these weight loss wonder cures are credible or not. After all these are commercial companies out to make money, and if they are successful they will lose customers.

Chapter 9

Dietary Supplements

Supplements whether they are vitamins, minerals or herbs play an important role in helping you maintain good health. It is a recognised fact that we no longer get all the nutrients from the foods we eat due to intensive farming practices, overuse of pesticides and fertilisers as well as the way food is processed and stored. So to make up the dietary shortfall you could supplement with a multivitamin and multi mineral supplement. When considering a supplement regime, make sure that they are manufactured from natural sources, not synthetic ones. Remember, synthetic supplements have no "life" in them.

Here is a short list for you to consider which could help to protect you against heart disease, high blood pressure & stroke:

B Complex Vitamins

B Complex provides the body with B vitamins which are critical for maintaining healthy functioning of the nervous system and for reducing the effects of stress upon the body. B vitamins are water soluble, and any excess is naturally excreted from the body, not stored, making continual replacement vital. All B vitamins work together this is why they are in a "complex" form.

Certain B Complex vitamins such as Choline which is derived from lecithin may prove beneficial for cardiovascular diseases, and inositol which is also found in lecithin is a complex form of fatty acid. Multiple reports promote inositol as a natural tranquiliser which alleviates anxiety and encourages sleep.

Vitamin C

According to the Journal of the American College of Nutrition, evidence overwhelmingly points to the value of vitamin C in maintaining health and preventing cancer, cardiovascular diseases and cataracts.

Vitamin C is a water soluble vitamin that must be obtained from dietary sources, and constantly replenished. Vitamin C helps form red blood cells and is necessary for the functioning of other nutrients in the body, such as intestinal absorption of iron which is significantly increased by sufficient levels of vitamin C.

Large quantities of vitamin C are found in the adrenal glands, as adequate amounts are essential for the creation of adrenalin. Adrenal ascorbic acid is quickly used up during periods of stress and anxiety.

Research done at *Cornell University* has shown that taking vitamin C along with rutin (a bioflavonoid) and vitamin A, reduces the chances of having a stroke by 75%. *Washington University* conducted a separate study which confirmed these findings.

Vitamin E with Selenium

Vitamin E is one of the most popular antioxidant vitamins. Studies have shown that men and women with high intakes of vitamin E have less coronary artery disease. Results from the *Cambridge Heart Antioxidant Study* found that taking 400IU—800IU of vitamin E daily reduced the risk of nonfatal heart attacks by 77 percent in patients with atherosclerosis. Vitamin E is also useful in reducing high blood pressure, and one of its constituents—tocotrienols may be effective in the fight against arteriosclerosis which is one of the major causes of a heart attack and stroke. Selenium is an antioxidant trace mineral that works with vitamin E. Low levels of selenium have been associated with an increased risk of cardiovascular disease.

Omega-3 EPA

An essential fatty acid from "oily" fish such as mackerel, salmon, sardines and tuna, plays an important role in keeping fats mobile in the blood stream. Research shows that a deficiency of Omega-3 Fatty Acids is linked to an increased risk of death from coronary heart disease.

The *American Heart Association* now recommends that anyone with coronary heart disease should consume approximately 1,000mg per day of "oily" fish or as an EPA supplement.

Studies suggest that a higher intake of EPA reduces the risk of cardiovascular disease which includes coronary heart disease, stroke and high blood pressure.

Flax Seed Oil

An essential fatty acid from plant sources, which contains Omega-3 EFA and Omega-6 EFA. Essential Fatty Acids are not produced by the body, and must be obtained from the diet. A deficiency of EFAs can lead to cardiovascular disease amongst other things. Numerous studies show that EFA supplementation improves an arteriosclerosis condition, helps lower blood pressure, restricts the formation of blood clots, and reduces cholesterol and triglycerides (blood fats).

Lecithin

Although it is a fatty substance, lecithin acts as a fat emulsifier, breaking down cholesterol and fat and helping to prevent these substances from sticking to the walls of arteries and vital organs. Lecithin causes fats, such as cholesterol to be dispersed in water and be removed from the body. Lecithin is known to help prevent arteriosclerosis and protect the body against heart disease. Lecithin is also important for memory function. One of its constituents acetyl choline is involved in the formation of the memory neurotransmitter acetylcholine.

Co Enzyme Q10 (CoQ10)

A naturally occurring nutrient found in nearly every cell of the human body. However, as we age production declines. Also diet, certain medications and lifestyle can affect body levels. It is essential for good heart health, as research has consistently confirmed there is a strong correlation between the severity of heart failure and low blood and tissue levels of CoQ10

Hawthorn Berries

Known as the heart herb for its many benefits as a heart tonic. Studies confirm traditional use of hawthorn berries to strengthen and normalise the heartbeat, prevent and reduce heart arrhythmias, and guard the heart against oxygen deficiency, as well as enhancing coronary circulation.

Hawthorn berries decreases high blood pressure by reducing heart output and enlarging peripheral blood vessels.

Ginkgo Biloba

An antioxidant herb that is one of the most popular prescription medications in both Germany and France, due to its many health benefits. Ginkgo Biloba contains bioflavonoids which are effective at reducing platelet aggregation (reduces blood platelets sticking together), as well as helping prevent cardiovascular diseases, such as atherosclerosis. It works well with hawthorn berries, and is often combined in herbal preparations.

Garlic

Garlic has been shown to treat a variety of circulatory disorders. Garlic inhibits platelet aggregation, it also helps in the breakdown and production of fibrin which is a clotting protein linked to heart disease and stroke. Garlic is excellent at lowering high blood pressure and helps lower serum levels of cholesterol and triglycerides (blood fats).

Remember whether it is your heart, high blood pressure or a stroke, prevention is better than cure. Sometimes it does not require major changes in diet and lifestyle to obtain significant health benefits, and you will feel better, have more energy and have a better quality of life.

Your health is in your own hands—so take good care of yourself.

Chapter 9

Detoxing

I am sure that you have heard of detoxing, maybe you have done a detox or colon cleanse yourself. Detoxing is important for eliminating toxic material from the body to ensure that your body is not carrying around a load of waste material.

So what are toxins, and where do they come from? Toxins take two forms (external and internal) and impact various parts of the body.

The external part comprises what we breathe in and what we eat and drink—usually a Western diet which is high in fats, sugars and chemicals and low in fiber. Other factors include: a lack of exercise, constipation, use of various medications as well as other lifestyle choices.

The internal part comprises the metabolic by-products of the diet. When the body digests food it creates toxic wastes. When the body is in healing and repairing mode it creates toxic wastes. If you experience negative emotions like anger and stress the body will create toxins.

These poisons build up in the colon, liver, kidneys and blood, in addition to causing inflammation in joint tissue which can lead to arthritis. Usually the early visible sign of toxins is when an eruption occurs on the surface of the skin. This can be in the form of pimples, blackheads, puss spots and other skin conditions.

Longer term, major health issues could arise such as chronic fatigue, depression, diabetes, heart, kidney and liver disease or cancer. Premature aging could also be a concern.

All these toxic factors impact the immune system which is the body's protection mechanism against disease. When the immune system is not working properly, it is then unable to protect the body against airborne invaders which enter through the nose, mouth and skin as well as metabolic changes within the body's structure.

Parasites and worms are often present when there is a toxic buildup in the body. These "invaders" are not your friends, and are only too happy to reside—usually in your colon, when a toxic environment is present. To help eradicate parasites and worms, various drug treatments are available which may be prescribed by your doctor, as well as more natural alternatives in the form of herbal remedies, which have been used for centuries to treat this problem.

Herbal detoxing involves purchasing herbal products either from a health food store or on the Internet. Several of these have their own celebrity followers. Some of these involve using various fruits and vegetables which you probably already have in your kitchen.

Whichever detoxing program you decide to use, before commencing , it is important to discuss this with your doctor to make sure what you propose doing is right for you. This is especially important if you are pregnant or breast feeding, or if you have any prior medical conditions and/or are taking any type of medication. It is important to ensure that any herbal remedies you propose taking do not conflict with any of your medications.

Chapter 10

How To Do A Detox

Human beings are mobile depositories for literally hundreds of different chemicals and toxins that in this modern age have become part of our homes and offices, so says the *Environmental Protection Agency (EPA)*, whose statements have been backed up by the majority of naturopathic doctors.

According to the *EPA* the air in our homes is more toxic than the air outside—even than in inner cities. This is mainly due to the fact that homes have become more airtight to improve the efficiency of air conditioning and heating systems; and that is not all, we are also bringing more cleaning chemicals into our homes as well.

Detoxing can take various forms from a simple colon cleanse to fasting and making significant changes to lifestyle choices. The body is a remarkable living thing, in that it has the ability to heal itself when given adequate nutrients and the tools it needs to do the job.

Sadly, the average Western diet is lacking in these nutrients and many synthetically manufactured vitamin and mineral supplements aren't always as bioavailable to the body as they should be. Bioavailable means that the supplements should be available to the body in much the same way that nutrients from food are.

A detoxification program basically means cleansing the body of toxins and chemicals that prevents it from maintaining optimum health. By expelling impurities—or helping the body to clear these impurities from the blood, liver, kidneys and intestines, every cell of the body will be improved. A detox program will enable the organs of the body to rest during a fastening process, thus stimulating the liver, promoting elimination, improving circulation and providing optimum fuel to the body through the addition of healthy nutrients.

The initial step in a detox process is to lighten the load on your body. During the detox, it is important to eliminate alcohol, coffee, cigarettes and refined sugars as well as saturated fats. All of these things are toxic to the body and provide obstacles in the healing process. It is also important to either eliminate or minimize the use of chemical based cleaners in the home in addition to personal care products which are ingested into the body through the skin and mucous membranes.

Additionally, it's important to look at other products in the home that are derived from plastic sources. An example of this is plastic containers made from polyvinyl chloride which releases toxic chemicals into the atmosphere. Another example is lead, although this is not so widely used today. However, in past decades lead in gasoline contributed to high levels of lead in the bones of women over the age of 40. To counteract any lead particles that may migrate into the bloodstream women should ensure they get adequate amounts of calcium, magnesium, and vitamin D, as well as a implementing a regular exercise program which will help to decrease the incidence of osteoporosis, also known as brittle bone disease.

It is also a good idea to dispense with the use of air fresheners in the home. While they may give off a nice scent, they are in fact filled with neurotoxins that have the effect of coating the inside of the nose which makes it difficult for you to "smell"—in reality, they don't really eliminate odors. It is far preferable to use natural alternatives such as: opening windows, placing some beautiful plants in the home or office, and make sure you empty the garbage cans frequently.

Drinking a minimum of 4 pints of filtered water each day will help to stimulate the kidneys, liver and digestive system to work more effectively. This will also help to boost your metabolism and accelerate the elimination of toxins from the body. Including other foods such as brown rice, herbal teas, garlic, lemons, cabbage and onions in your diet will also assist your body to eliminate built-up toxins.

It is also important to add more fiber to your diet. Statistics show that the average American diet is badly lacking in adequate fiber; this has the effect of increasing toxic build-up in the cells as well as an increased incidence of constipation. Also organically grown fruits and vegetables will assist in elimination and cleansing of the colon. In addition, you can help to improve the function of the liver by using various herbs such Milk Thistle and Dandelion Root as well as drinking green tea. Increasing your levels of vitamins C. will assist the body in producing glutathione—an antioxidant which is another compound that helps to eliminate toxins and prevent premature aging, in addition to warding off chronic disease.

Stress is often a major factor in everyday life, but it is also another toxin to the body. Stress has a negative impact on the liver and kidneys, as well as the circulatory system; it can cause increased hypertension (high blood pressure). All of these problems can be precursors to more serious health issues. By reducing the stress in your life and promoting more positive emotional feelings you will go a long way in helping to detoxifying your lifestyle.

You may consider beginning your toxic detoxifying process by going on a fast. Nutritionists believe that fasting for 24 hours every two weeks or one month is actually very healthy for the body. In modern times we actually very rarely go hungry, but in past centuries when we had to forage for all our food, days may go by with nothing to eat at all. This in effect was a natural fasting process, and we can replicate this today by doing a modern-day fast involving drinking filtered water and juices made from organic fruits and vegetables. Doing this, you'll rest your liver and intestines enabling them to work more efficiently.

Did you know that sweat and perspiration is used by the body as a means of eliminating toxins? You can assist the body's toxin elimination process with the use of saunas, exercise and hot showers which all have the effect of eliminating waste material from the body. Dry brushing your skin can also assist in removing toxins through the pores. In fact, special brushes are available for this purpose from various natural product stores.

Removing excess chemicals and toxins from the body will have a very positive impact on your overall health and well-being.

Chapter 11

Good Colon Health

Consuming the typical Western diet means that many Americans suffer from poor colon health, and unfortunately many are not aware of it. The condition of the stool that is excreted gives a good indication of the health of the colon. A good stool pattern requires the ability to eliminate two or three stools that are formed each day. The first stool which should also be the longest should be expelled in the morning; a stool half of this size should be expelled later the same day. When eliminating stools there should be no straining involved; the stool should be expelled without any effort.

Constipation causes a build-up of stool in the colon wall, which does not bode well for good health. This build-up of fecal matter which may have been there for many years, can cause inflammation in the colon, with the result that a decaying effect is triggered, which causes a toxic build-up causing other tissues and organs of the body to be affected, as it travels throughout the bloodstream. This condition can cause the intestinal wall to leech bacteria and viruses into the bloodstream, which can result in various chronic illnesses in the body.

In fact the colon is one of the major areas in the body where toxins reside, and if it is left untreated, then, it becomes a breeding ground for all kinds of unfriendly bacteria, parasites, worms and amoeba like structures all of which have one purpose—to do your body harm. They are not your friends.

Many people who undertake a colon cleanse often lose as much as 7–9 pounds in body weight. This is all impacted toxic matter that has been purged out of the system, along with any parasites that reside there.

It is not difficult to maintain good colon health. One of the most effective things you can do is to increase your fiber intake, as well as eating more fruits and vegetables. Fiber is one of the best ways to help prevent constipation. The ideal daily dietary fiber intake should be 38 grams for men and 25 grams for women.

This figure is based on adults less than 50 years of age. If you are over 50 then men should consume 30 grams of fiber each day and women 21 grams. It is also important to consume at least eight glasses of filtered water each day to help the fiber work more effectively, and in addition, it also helps prevent a hard stool which can result in constipation.

In addition, doing a regular exercise program at least 3 to 4 times a week for 30 minutes each time will also help to stimulate all your body systems, which can also have a positive effect on colon health.

Laxatives should be used sparingly and not as a regular daily occurrence. Additionally, do not ignore your body's urge to have a bowel movement. If you do, this can cause a lazy colon which can lead to constipation.

If you think you are constipated then you could try drinking prune juice or eating prunes before deciding on laxatives. And also remember to add fiber and water to your diet.

If you have persistent constipation it is probably a good idea to consult your doctor to determine there are no other underlying health issues which may be causing the problem.

Chapter 12

What About Doing A Colon Cleanse

The purpose of colon cleansing is to help reduce bloating, constipation and fatigue. There are two schools of thought regarding this subject. Those in favor believe that colon cleansing has significant health benefits, whilst many doctors on the other hand take a different view. Doctors often recommend a colon cleanse in preparation for a medical examination or surgery, but don't recommend it on a regular basis.

One of the purposes of the colon is to absorb water and sodium to help maintain the body's electrolyte balance; the danger is that regular colon cleansing can disrupt this balance, with the result that salt depletion can occur as well as dehydration. If done over a long period of time, this can lead to heart failure, anemia and malnutrition.

Many healthcare professionals recommend colon cleansing as the result of the majority of people eating a standard Western diet which is common in the US as well as many parts of Europe. This diet is high in saturated fat, meat, polyunsaturated fats and processed foods.

The problem with this type of diet is that it exposes the colon and intestines to decomposing foods for a longer period of time. This rotting food exposes an individual to a greater risk of developing intestinal diseases. Those people who enjoy a vegetarian diet have a reduced risk for developing an intestinal illness since the food they eat moves through the intestines much more quickly because animal fats are not included in the diet.

There are two main kinds of colon cleansing. The first comprises a powder or liquid supplements which works from the top down. These can be bought from health food stores, supermarkets or on the Internet. The second is colonic irrigation or hydrotherapy which involves an enema to flush out the lower intestines with water. Holistic practitioners believe that if the colon is not kept clean, fecal waste material will build up, which will then harden and decrease the absorption of nutrients into the body. Also, these unwanted toxins and chemicals may have a negative impact on the integrity of the intestinal wall.

As these toxins and chemicals build up in the intestines, there is a danger that a build-up of bad bacteria or viruses can occur, which may cause a leaking of these viruses or bacteria into the abdominal cavity or bloodstream. Add all this together, and we have a scenario where we could have a seriously compromised intestinal system.

Using a colon cleansing program may not just involve the colon but the entire intestinal tract. This approach may assist the body to work more efficiently, and at the same time give you more energy in addition to ridding the system of all the toxins, chemicals, bad bacteria and viruses.

One of the most effective colon cleanses involves including a high fiber diet possibly using psyllium husks that is low in fat and high in vitamin D. Incorporating a regular exercise program is also beneficial as it helps to move waste materials through the colon, ready for elimination.

A high fiber diet also reduces the risk of constipation. However, it is always important to remember that high fiber diets also need adequate amounts of filtered water—ideally, eight glasses per day. This will help to keep your body hydrated, as well as helping the fiber work more effectively.

To detoxify your body using colon cleanses is a personal decision for you to make. Detoxing however, is only part of the story. You also need to possibly make other lifestyle changes as well. These could include incorporating an exercise program as well as making choices in the type of foods you eat. And never forget the all-important daily liquid—ideally filtered water— your body needs to keep hydrated as well. All of these things assist your body in performing its billions of daily functions to help you enjoy your lifestyle and keep you healthy.

Chapter 13

Consider A Cleansing Diet

A cleansing diet is an excellent way to purge your body of toxins or undigested food items. There are various cleansing diets available each with their own approach to detoxification.

Some cleansing diets are based on only eating one of two different types of foods. Some are based on only drinking liquids but no solid foods at all, while still allowing a person to eat several types of food. Then there are cleansing programs which feature various herbal combinations. So you can see there is a wide choice available so it is important for each individual to choose a cleansing diet program that they will feel comfortable with.

Every person is exposed to chemical toxins as they go about their daily life. Toxins take many forms: some are residual products of the foods that have been eaten, whilst others are classed as environmental toxins which are airborne and are breathed in. As toxins are invisible, they are often little thought about, but it is important to purge them from the body. It is a good idea to do a cleansing program at least twice a year which will help the body systems function more effectively.

As mentioned above, one type of cleansing diet involves only drinking bottled water and freshly squeezed juices. In reality, you may not wish to continue with a cleansing diet for a long period of time due to its intensity. An adequate amount of time is usually between 3 to 7 days. Of note, this type of cleanse is sometimes used prior to your doctor performing tests on your lower and upper gastrointestinal tract.

Some individuals use a vegan type diet as a cleansing program. This involves eating natural fruits and vegetables. All forms of meat, dairy products and carbohydrates are eliminated on this type of diet. Drinks consist of either water or freshly squeezed juices.

While on a cleansing diet if you start to feel unwell then you should start to eat something a little more substantial. It is not necessary to eat a full course meal, but only to eat something that is a bit more filling. It is also important, and indeed advisable to take a multivitamin supplement every day to make up for vitamin and mineral shortfalls in the diet whilst you're on a cleansing diet program. In addition, it is also important to drink plenty of filtered or bottled still water, and also get adequate amounts of rest and sleep.

In years gone by people rarely ate three large meals each day, as is often normal practice today. For example, farmers often ate a large breakfast and dinner but skipped lunch because they were busy in the fields all day. In addition, because of their physical activity they burnt a lot of the calories off each day. As another example, native tribes whose life revolved around hunting and gathering would frequently go for several days without food when it couldn't be found. This type of eating plan allowed the body to cleanse itself naturally.

When you are near the end of your cleansing diet program you should start to gradually introduce a variety of foods back into your body in small amount at a time. It is not a good idea to introduce everything back all at once as this could put your body into shock mode. Remember, your body has been deprived of its natural food intake for several days so it will need some time to readjust back to normal again. Eating small meals is advisable as your body readjusts back to normal. The last thing your body needs is to be weighed down with a heavy caloric intake again.

To have your body free of toxins is a worthwhile goal to aim for. A body that is loaded with toxins cannot work effectively, and it can be exposed to various ailments and health conditions if it is left in this state over time.

Chapter 14

Consult Your Doctor or a Naturopathic Doctor

In this book I have given you some dietary supplement and herbal product suggestions that have been used historically by herbalists and naturopaths for many years, but no suggested dosage requirements, or contra-indications.

The reason for this is that everyone is different. One person may need more of a particular product than the next person. Also, a particular product may suit one person, but not another.

Therefore I feel it is extremely important that you consult your doctor or a naturopathic doctor before commencing any supplement or herbal program, or changing your diet.

Additionally, you may be taking prescription medications for various health conditions which will, or could, have a negative impact on your health if you introduce vitamin or mineral supplements or an herbal program. Never take chances with your health.

I know that many doctors are not supportive of using a natural traditional route for health care. If your doctor feels this way and you would like to consider a more natural approach, then change your doctor and find one who is more supportive to your requirements.

Reference Tables

The major causes of death in the USA, Canada, part of the UK (England and Wales) and Australia. You can find further information by going to each country's statistics website. The downloads are free! These are the latest tables available in 2021.

USA	**2020**	
Total Deaths (Male and Female)	3,358,814	100.00%
Heart Disease	690,892	20.57%
Cancer	598,932	17.83%
Covid-19	345,323	10.28%
Unintentional Injuries	192,176	5.72%
Stroke	159,050	4.74%
Respiratory System Diseases	151,637	4.51%
Alzheimer's Disease	133,382	3.97%
Diabetes Mellitus	101,106	3.01%
Influenza and Pneumonia	53,495	1.59%
Kidney Disease	52,260	1.56%
All Other Causes	880,561	26.22%

Canada	**2019**	
Total Deaths (Male and Female)	284,082	100.00%
Cancer	81,913	28.83%
Cardiovascular Disease	71,646	25.22%
Respiratory System Diseases	16,792	5.91%
Unintentional Accidents	13,746	4.84%
Abnormal Clinical/Laboratory Findings	8,085	2.85%
Diabetes Mellitus	6,912	2.43%
Influenza & Pneumonia	6,893	2.43%
Alzheimer's Disease	6,166	2.17%
Nephritis	3,767	1.33%
Chronic Liver Disease	3,662	1.29%
All Other Causes	64,500	22.70%

England and Wales	**2018**	
Total Deaths (Male and Female)	541,589	100.00%
Neoplasms (Cancer)	149,868	27.67%
Circulatory System Diseases	132,233	24.41%
Respiratory System Diseases	76,728	14.17%
Mental & Behavorial Disorders	50,804	9.38%
Digestive System Diseases	25,699	4.74%
External Causes Of Morbadity & Mortality	23,117	4.27%
Alzheimer's Disease	19,864	3.67%
Nervous System Diseases: Exc Alzheimer's	15,754	2.91%
Urinary System Diseases	8,846	1.63%
Diabetes Mellitus	6,349	1.18%
All Other Causes	32,327	5.97%

Australia	**2019**	
Total Deaths (Male and Female)	169,301	100.00%
Cancer	48,642	28.73%
Circulatory System Diseases	43,249	25.55%
Respiratory System Diseases	16,275	9.61%
External Causes Of Morbidity & Mortality	11,794	6.97%
Mental & Behavorial Disorders	11,033	6.52%
Endocrine & Metabolic Diseases	7,101	4.19%
Digestive System Diseases	6,413	3.79%
Diabetes Mellitus	4,967	2.94%
Alzheimers Disease	4,578	2.70%
Urinary System Diseases	4,035	2.38%
All Other Causes	11,214	6.62%

Do You Live In a European Union Country

Of particular concern in Europe. In 2011 the European Union introduced the Herbal Medicines Directive which means the herbal industry has been all but destroyed by a draconian law which has all but banned the supply of herbal products within the European Union.

The excuse for issuing this directive is "*to ensure public safety with regard to herbal products*". I would have thought that something that has been used safely for hundreds (and in some cases thousands) of years would be safe for the public to take.

Many herbal products have been classified, not for use in food preparation (i.e. for cooking or garnishing purposes) but as "medicines" and a company now needs a license in order to sell them to the public. The cost of the license is in the order of $150,000 per herbal product. Yes, you read that correctly, $150,000 per herbal product.

Say you are a manufacturer and have just a small range of just 20 herbal products that is going to cost you $3,000,000 in license fees, before you can sell anything. Very few manufacturers have that kind of money to waste on licenses for something that has been used safely for all those years. Therefore, it is hard luck if you live in a European Union country

And there is more! In early 2013 without warning or any consultation, Milk Thistle was banned from sale in the UK. It is now classed as a medicine and needs a licence in order for a manufacturer to sell it. Why? Milk Thistle has been used safely for hundreds of years to detoxify the liver. This to me seems like wanton vandalism for the sake of it.

All these new laws are going to do is drive the supply of these safe, natural herbal products underground. With the power of modern communications and the Internet, all you have to do is spend a little time seeking out those herbal products you require from sources outside Europe. Many suppliers in other parts of the world—and especially in the United States—will be more than happy to supply you, and will ship their products internationally. As the saying goes—where there's a will there's a way!!

About The Author

Brian B Jacques started in business at a young age, and over the ensuing years, he has developed several very successful businesses. But his main interest for the past 40 years has been in natural health research and publishing.

Brian has presented seminars worldwide on such diverse subjects as Health Related issues, Motivation and Personal Development. In addition he has written numerous books, newsletters and articles on these subjects.

His very popular series of Mini Health Books has circulated widely around the world, and many more titles are in preparation.

Brian is a highly motivated individual, so much so that in 1985 he received a UK Industrial Society award for his work in the Motivation and Personal Development fields.

Brian has the following mottos:

- If something does not work out for you, then don't give up, but keep trying, trying, trying until finally you succeed.
- Success or failure in any endeavor is in your own hands.

Brian and his wife divide their time between East Yorkshire, UK and Florida, USA.

www.ingramcontent.com/pod-product-compliance
Ingram Content Group UK Ltd.
Pitfield, Milton Keynes, MK11 3LW, UK
UKHW022010190726
13853UKWH00004B/1851